Crazy Egg

Chicken Egg Cookbook

30 Delicious Recipes

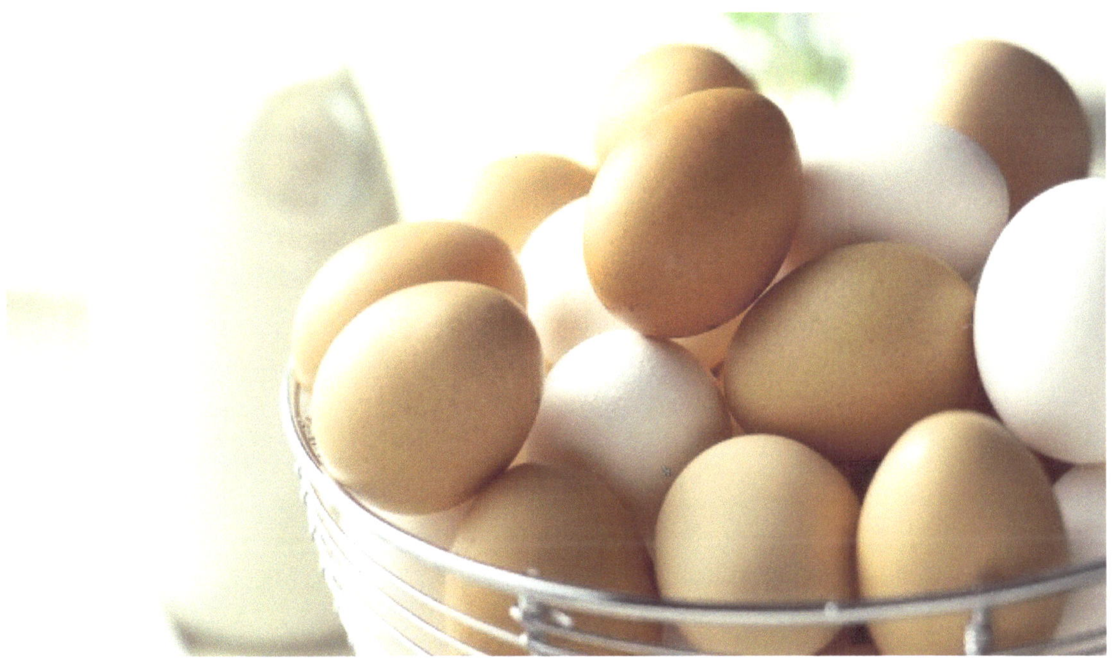

Content

Introduction

Eggs are rich in protein, vitamins, and minerals. Yes, we all know that but did you know that it controls cholesterol too? Which means that if you intake egg, you will not be having any blood pressure problem in your later stage of life. Eggs are known to be very versatile because they provide you with unlimited nutrients to different parts of the body. There are so many ways of cooking eggs and adding them to the recipes which will mesmerize you.

Since the chicken came into the being, eggs have been enjoyed as nourishment in history. It has known to be the reason for fertility and provide important nutrients with folic acids. Females who are pregnant are recommended to have the intake of egg because of the folic acid which is required for the development process to start. There are different types of eggs available in the market but mostly chicken eggs are used for cooking and eating all around the world. For baking purposes, only chicken eggs are preferred because they provide you with excellent results.

Other eggs may include duck, goose and quail eggs which are eaten by rare percentage all around the world.

Eggs are not expensive which is why they are found in every household. No matter they eat it daily or not, it is found everywhere. The white part of the egg contains iron, copper, zinc along with lecithin. It is the same compound which is found in mayonnaise as well.

Here are a few tips to make sure that you will get that desirable egg dish that you are craving for.

1. For health conscious people organic egg is the best.
2. There are many ways to cook hard-boiled egg, but the easiest way to do this is by putting the eggs into boiling water and cook for 10 minutes.
3. When cooking soft-boiled eggs, simmer covered for about 5-7 minutes before serving time to get that runny or barely set egg-yolk.
4. If you want fluffy scrambled eggs, add a few tablespoons of milk then slightly tilt the bowl with eggs while beating constantly to allow some air bubbles to form, but do not overdo it.
5. When cooking omelets, allow the egg to cook and fully set at the bottom before adding the filling and gently flipping half of the egg to cover the filling.
6. Poaching egg is similar to frying an egg, but instead of oil you will use water to cook the egg. Normally, the white part of the egg gets solidified while the yolk remains to be runny.
7. To test for eggs freshness: Place uncooked egg in a bowl filled with water. If the egg stays on its side at the bottom, you'll know it is fresh. If the egg floats, it is no longer fresh and not safe to eat.
8. Using sliced vegetables such as onion and bell pepper, is perfect in making egg cups.

9. When buying eggs, they should be clean and free from cracks.

10. When storing eggs, don't remove them in their original packaging (egg tray) and place on the coldest part of the refrigerator. Not on the designed tray that you can find in the door.

11. Properly stored fresh or raw eggs can be kept up to 3-5 weeks. While, refrigerated leftover cooked eggs should be consumed within 3 days.

12. If you want to cut down on calories, fat, and cholesterol in your egg dishes you can substitute half of your egg requirement with egg whites (2 egg whites = 1 egg).

Thank you for downloading this book!
It is my sincere hope that it will answer your questions on Egg recipes!

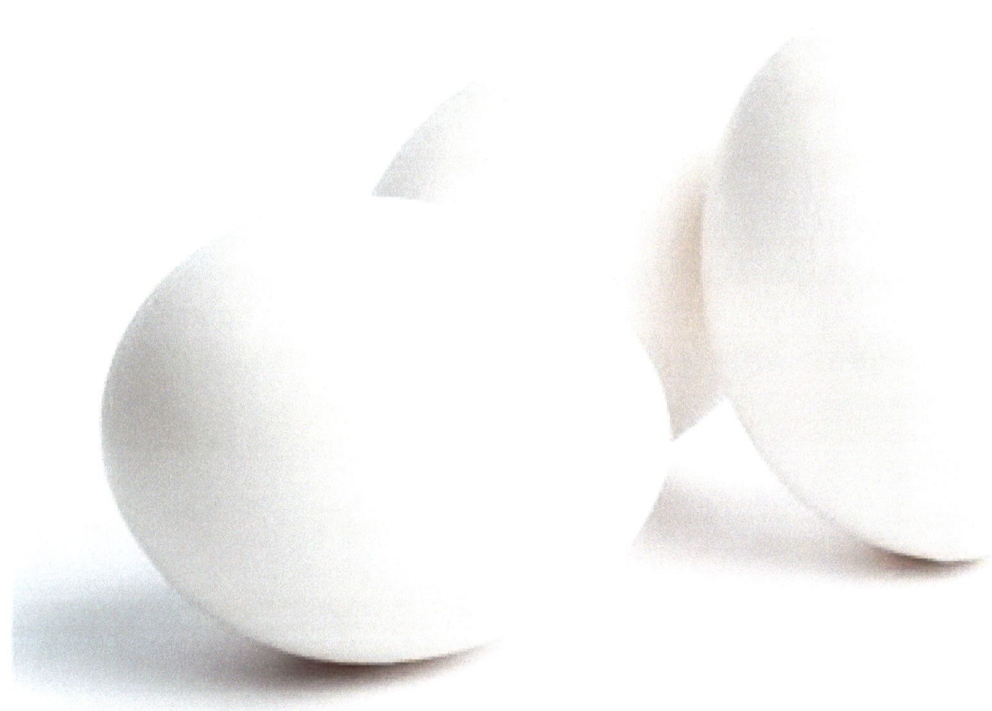

Chapter 1. Scrambled

Scrambled Egg with Minced Chicken and Herb

Treat yourself this weekend with this great tasting scrambled eggs with minced chicken, rosemary, and thyme.

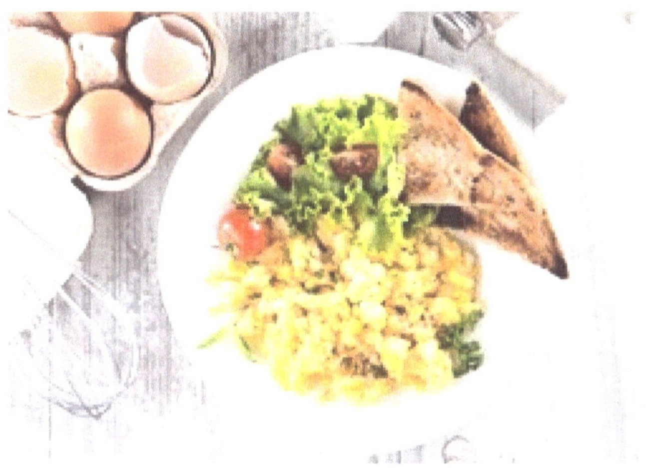

Serves: 4
Preparation Time: 10 minutes

Ingredients

- 5 large eggs
- 2 tablespoons milk
- 1 tablespoon vegetable oil
- 2 cloves garlic, minced
- 8 oz. chicken breast fillet, minced
- ¼ teaspoon dried rosemary
- ¼ teaspoon dried thyme
- salt and freshly ground black pepper

Directions

1. Beat eggs and milk in a medium bowl.
2. Heat oil in a large non-stick pan or skillet over medium-high heat. Stir-fry garlic for 1 minute.
3. Add minced chicken, rosemary, and thyme. Cook for 3 minutes or until browned, stirring occasionally.
4. Pour beaten egg mixture into the pan. Cook, stirring constantly for 2-3 minutes or to desired doneness.
5. Season with salt srad pepper, to taste.
6. Serve and enjoy!

Scrambled Egg with Feta and Parsley

Start your day with this simple yet delicious scrambled egg recipe for breakfast!

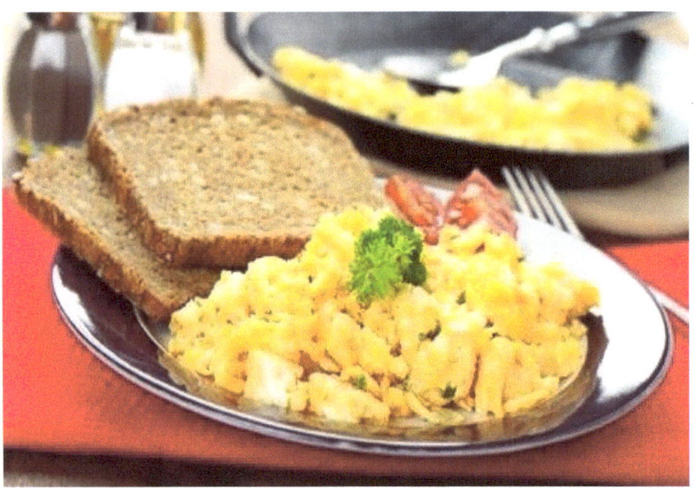

Serves: 3-4
Preparation Time: 10 minutes

Ingredients

- 4 large eggs
- 2 egg whites
- 2 tablespoons milk
- 1 tablespoon butter
- 1 shallot, chopped
- 1 clove garlic, minced
- ½ cup cottage cheese
- 2 tablespoons fresh parsley, chopped freshly ground black pepper

Directions

1. Whisk eggs and milk in a medium bowl.
2. Melt butter in a large non-stick pan or skillet over medium-high heat. Stir-fry shallot and garlic for 1 minute.
3. Pour beaten egg mixture into the pan. Add cottage cheese and parsley.
4. Cook, stirring constantly for 2-3 minutes or to desired doneness.
5. Season with pepper, to taste.
6. Serve and enjoy!

Scrambled Egg with Mushroom and Cheese

Enjoy this healthy and filling breakfast recipe with eggs, mushrooms, and cheese.

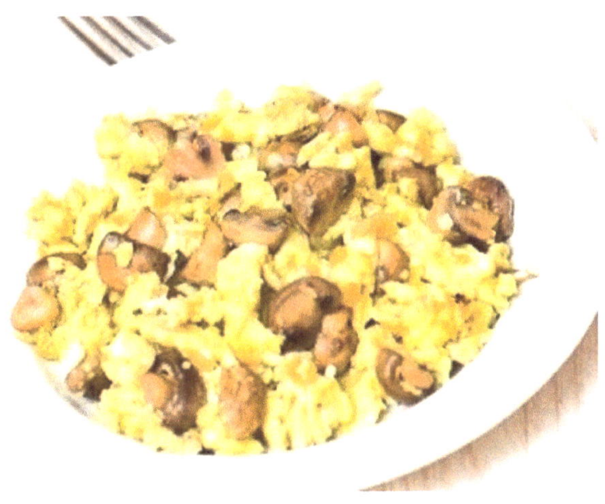

Serves: 4
Preparation Time: 10 minutes

Ingredients

- 3 large eggs
- 2 egg whites
- 2 tablespoons milk
- 1 tablespoon vegetable oil
- 2 cloves garlic, minced
- ½ cup button mushrooms, sliced
- ¼ teaspoon dried sage
- ¼ cup cheddar cheese, grated
- salt and freshly ground black pepper

Directions

1. Beat eggs and milk in a medium bowl.
2. Heat oil in a large non-stick pan or skillet over medium-high heat. Stir-fry garlic for 1 minute.
3. Add button mushrooms and sage. Cook for 2-3 minutes, stirring occasionally.
4. Pour beaten egg mixture into the pan.
5. Add cheese. Cook, stirring constantly for 2-3 minutes or to desired doneness.
6. Season with salt and pepper, to taste.
7. Serve and enjoy!

Scrambled Egg with Onion and Tomato

Serve this awesome scrambled eggs with toasts for a filling breakfast or brunch in 10 minutes or less!

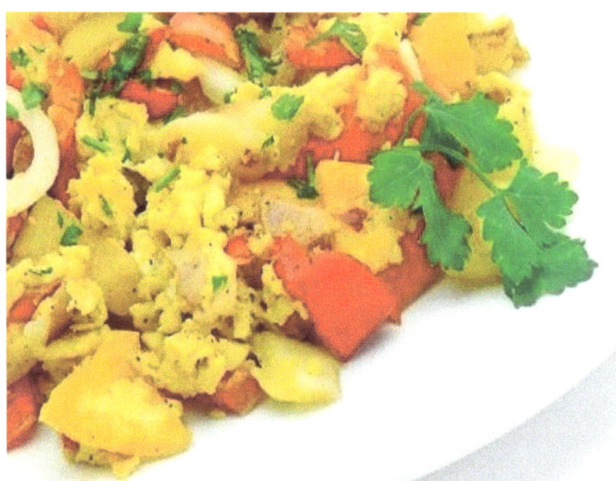

Serves: 3-4
Preparation Time: 10 minutes

Ingredients

- 5 large eggs
- ¼ cup milk
- 1 tablespoon olive oil
- 1 large white onion, chopped
- 2 cloves garlic, minced
- 2 medium tomatoes, chopped
- 2 tablespoons fresh parsley
- salt and freshly ground black pepper

Directions

1. Whisk together eggs and milk in a medium bowl.
2. Heat oil in a large non-stick pan or skillet over medium-high heat. Stir-fry onion and garlic for 1 minute.
3. Add the tomatoes. Cook for 2-3 minutes, stirring occasionally.
4. Pour beaten egg mixture into the pan.
5. Add parsley. Cook, stirring constantly for 2-3 minutes or to desired doneness.
6. Season with salt and pepper, to taste.
7. Serve and enjoy!

Fluffy Scrambled Egg with Cheddar

This easy to make scrambled egg recipe with mayonnaise and cheddar is so creamy and fluffy!

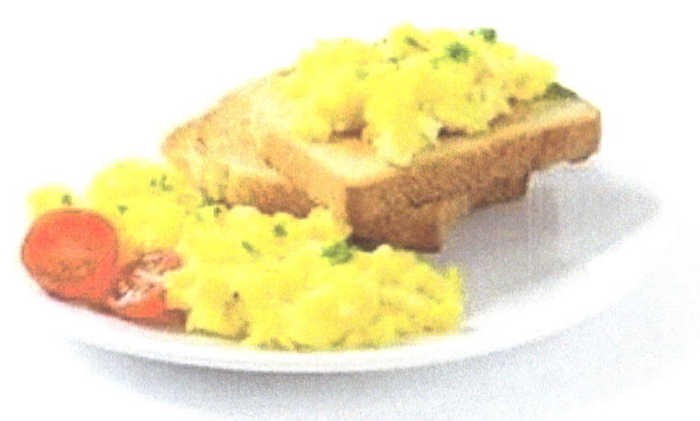

Serves: 3-4
Preparation Time: 10 minutes

Ingredients

- 3 large eggs
- 3 egg whites
- 2 tablespoons mayonnaise
- 1 tablespoon milk
- 1 tablespoon olive oil
- 1 shallot, chopped
- ¼ cup cheddar cheese, grated
- 2 tablespoons green onions, chopped
- salt and freshly ground black pepper

Directions

1. Beat eggs, mayonnaise, and milk in a medium bowl.
2. Heat oil in a large non-stick pan or skillet over medium-high heat. Stir-fry shallot for 1 minute.
3. Pour the beaten egg mixture into the pan.
4. Add cheese and sprinkle with green onions. Cook, stirring constantly for 2-3 minutes or to your desired doneness.
5. Season with salt and pepper, to taste.
6. Serve and enjoy!

Chapter 2. Omelet

Easy Bean and Coriander Omellette

Grab a bite of this savory omelet with baked chili beans and coriander.

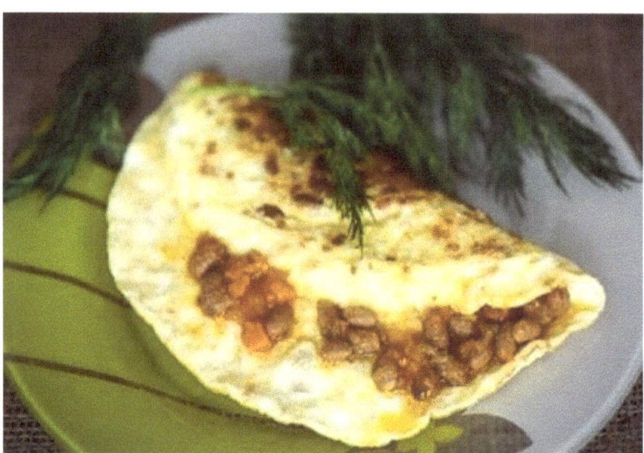

Serves: 2-3
Preparation Time: 10 minutes

Ingredients

- 4 medium eggs
- 1 Tbsp. butter
- 2/3 cup baked chili beans
- 1 teaspoon fresh coriander, chopped
- salt and freshly ground black pepper

Directions

1. Whisk the eggs and season with salt and pepper, to taste.
2. Heat butter in a non-stick pan over medium heat.
3. Pour egg and cook for about 2 minutes. Gently lift the edge of the egg mixture with a spatula, let uncooked egg mixture flow to the edges of the pan to cook. Cook for about 1-2 minutes.
4. Top half of the egg with baked chili and beans. Sprinkle with coriander. Slowly lift the egg to cover the bean filling. Cook further 1-2 minutes.
5. Transfer into a serving plate.
6. Serve and enjoy!

Herbed Salmon Tomato Omelette

This is a wonderful omelet recipe to serve your family any day of the week.

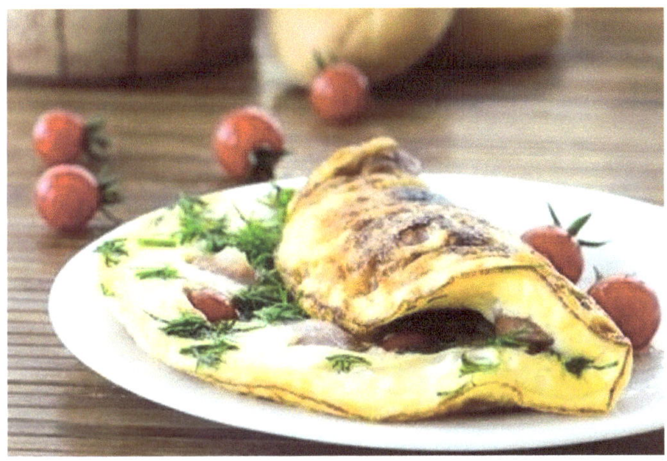

Serves: 2-3
Preparation Time: 10 minutes

Ingredients

- 4 medium eggs
- 2 tablespoons olive oil
- 1 shallot, thinly sliced
- 1 clove garlic, crushed
- ½ cup cherry tomatoes, halved
- 2 oz. smoked salmon, chopped
- 2 Tbsp. fresh parsley, chopped
- salt and freshly ground black pepper, to taste

Directions

1. Beat eggs and season with salt and pepper, to taste.
2. Heat 1 tablespoon oil in a non-stick pan over medium heat. Stir-fry shallot and garlic for 1 minute.
3. Add the cherry tomatoes and salmon. Cook for another 1-2 minutes. Transfer to a clean plate. Set aside.
4. In the same pan, heat remaining oil. Pour egg and cook for about 2 minutes. Gently lift the edge of the egg mixture with a spatula, let uncooked egg mixture flow to the edges of the pan to cook. Cook for about 1-2 minutes.
5. Top half of the egg with tomato-salmon mixture. Sprinkle with parsley. Gently lift the other side to cover the filling. Cook further 1-2 minutes.
6. Transfer into a serving dish.
7. Serve and enjoy!

Mediterranean Style Omelette

This Mediterranean-flavored omelet is sure to please.

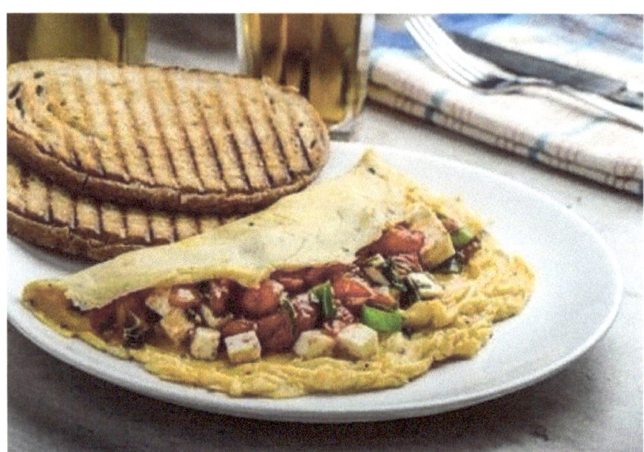

Serves: 2-3
Preparation Time: 15 minutes

Ingredients

- 4 medium eggs
- 2 Tbsp. olive oil
- 1 medium onion, chopped
- 1 clove garlic, crushed
- 1 medium tomato, diced
- 1 medium green bell pepper, diced
- ½ cup feta cheese, diced
- 2 tbsp. fresh basil, chopped salt and freshly ground black pepper, to taste

Directions

1. Beat the eggs and season with salt and pepper, to taste.
2. Heat 1 tablespoon oil in a non-stick pan over medium heat. Stir-fry onion and garlic for 1 minute.
3. Add the tomato and green bell pepper. Cook until soft, stirring frequently. Transfer to a plate and set aside.
4. Using the same pan, heat remaining oil. Pour egg and cook for about 2 minutes. Gently lift the edge of the egg mixture with a spatula, let uncooked egg mixture flow to the edges of the pan to cook. Cook for about 2 minutes.
5. Top half of the egg with tomato mixture, feta cheese, and basil. Gently lift the other side over the vegetable and feta filling. Cook further 1-2 minutes.
6. Slide omelet into a serving dish.
7. Serve and enjoy!

Pepper Broccoli and Cheese Omelette

This delightful omelet recipe with pepper, broccoli, mozzarella, and cheddar is a great way to get your kids to eat vegetables.

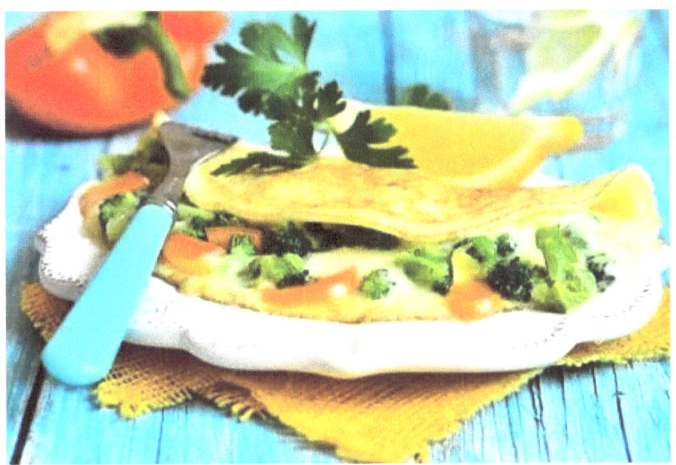

Serves: 2-3
Preparation Time: 15 minutes

Ingredients
- 4 medium eggs
- 2 tbsp. olive oil
- 1 medium shallot, chopped
- 1 medium red bell pepper
- 1 cup broccoli, coarsely chopped
- ¼ cup mozzarella cheese, diced
- 2 tbsp. cheddar cheese
- salt and freshly ground black pepper

Directions
1. Beat the eggs and season with salt and pepper, to taste.
2. Heat 1 tablespoon oil in a non-stick pan over medium heat. Stir-fry shallot for 1 minute.
3. Add the bell pepper and broccoli. Cook until soft, about 5 minutes, stirring frequently. Transfer to a plate and set aside.
4. Using the same pan, heat remaining oil. Pour egg and cook for about 2 minutes. Gently lift the edge of the egg mixture with a spatula, let uncooked egg mixture flow to the edges of the pan to cook. Cook for about 1-2 minutes.
5. Top half of the egg with vegetable mixture, mozzarella, and cheddar. Gently lift the other side to cover the vegetable and cheese filling. Cook further 1-2 minutes or until done.
6. Slide omelet into a serving dish. Garnish with fresh parsley.
7. Serve and enjoy!

Shrimp and Cheddar Omelette with Chives

This seafood omelet made with shrimp, cheddar, and chives is good to have any time of the day.

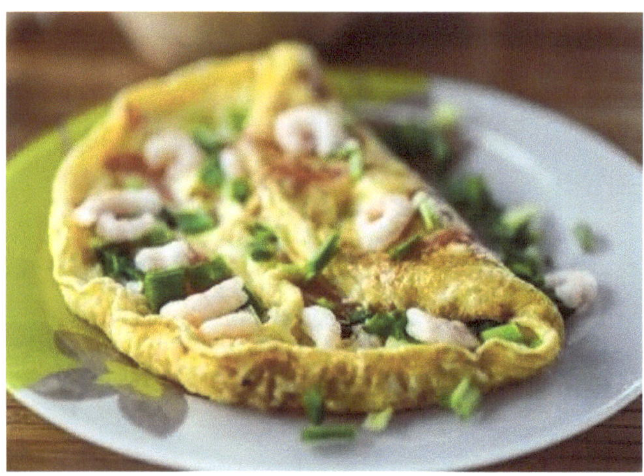

Serves: 2-3
Preparation Time: 20 minutes

Ingredients

- 4 medium eggs
- 2 Tbsp. olive oil
- 1 medium onion, chopped
- 1 clove garlic, crushed
- 3 oz. small shrimps, peeled and deveined
- ¼ cup chives, chopped
- salt and freshly ground black pepper, to taste

Directions

1. In a medium bowl, beat the eggs. Season with salt and pepper, to taste.
2. Heat 1 tablespoon oil in a non-stick pan over medium heat. Stir-fry onion and garlic for 1 minute.
3. Add the shrimps. Cook for 2-3 minutes, stirring constantly until it turned pink. Transfer to a plate and set aside.
4. Using the same pan, heat remaining oil. Pour egg and cook for about 2 minutes. Gently lift the edge of the egg mixture with a spatula, let uncooked egg mixture flow to the edges of the pan to cook. Cook for about 2 minutes.
5. Top half of the egg with shrimps. Sprinkle with chives. Gently lift the other side to cover the shrimp filling. Cook further 1-2 minutes.
6. Slide omelet into a serving dish.
7. Serve and enjoy!

Chapter 3. Boiled, Salads recipes

Twisty Egg Salad

You will love the taste of this pasta along with the vegetables and eggs ingredients.

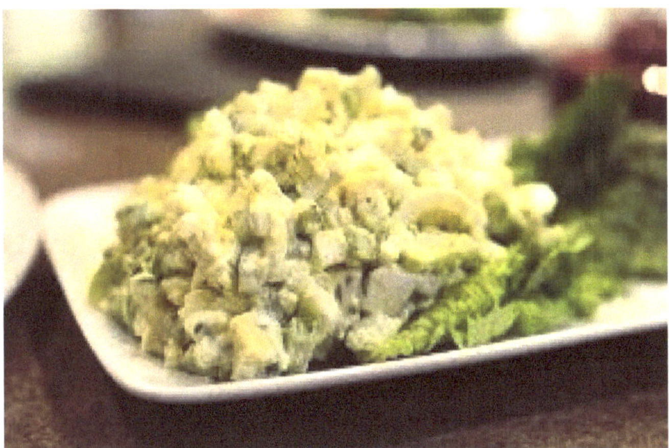

Serves: 2
Preparation Time: 15 minutes

Ingredients

- Pasta twists–2 cups
- Boiled eggs–2
- Celery sticks–2
- Red capsicum(sliced) –1
- Green onions(chopped) –2
- Parsley leaves2 cups
- Egg mayonnaise–2 tbsp.
- Wholegrain mustard–2 tbsp.
- Lemon juice–2 tbsp.

Directions

1. Boil the pasta twists for 10 minutes and rinse them when ready.
2. Add boiled eggs, celery sticks, red capsicum and green onion into the bowl.
3. Add oil into the pan and cook the mixture.
4. When done, add parsley, mayonnaise, mustard and lemon juice.
5. Mix well.
6. Mix both pasta and mixture into a large bowl.
7. When ready, serve. Enjoy!

Ultimate Cobb Salad with Poppy Seed Dressing

Packed with a variety of delicious ingredients, this filling salad makes a great summer lunch.

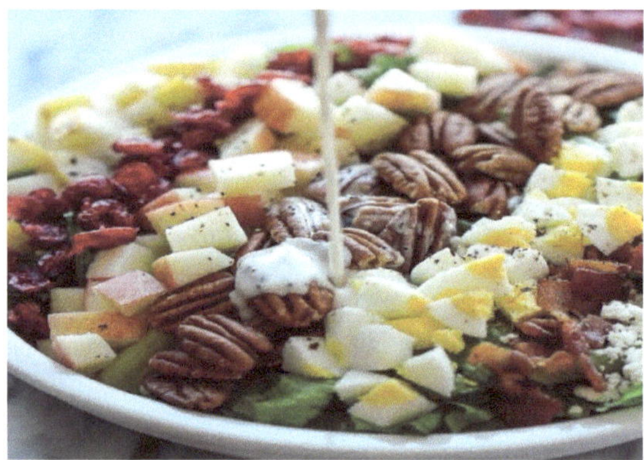

Serves: 4

Preparation Time: 20 minutes

Ingredients

Dressing

- ⅓ cup full-fat mayo
- ¼ cup whole milk
- 2 tbsp. sugar
- 1 tbsp. apple cider vinegar
- 1 tbsp. poppy seeds

Salad

- 4 rashers unsmoked bacon (diced)
- 6 cups lettuce of choice
- 2 hardboiled eggs (chopped)
- 1 red apple (chopped)
- 1 pear (chopped)
- ½ cup pecans (chopped)
- ⅓ cup dried pecans
- ⅓ cup goat cheese (crumbled)

Directions

1. Combine all dressing ingredients in a bowl, stir well and set aside.
2. Sauté the bacon pieces in a skillet over med-high heat, until crispy. Transfer to a plate and pat away any excess grease with kitchen paper. Set aside.
3. Into the base of a large salad bowl, make a bed of lettuce.
4. Arrange the remaining ingredients in rows on top of the lettuce and then drizzle over the poppy seed dressing.
5. Serve. Enjoy!

Egg Green Salad

Losing weight is not easy, this recipe will help your stomach filled along with providing essential nutrients.

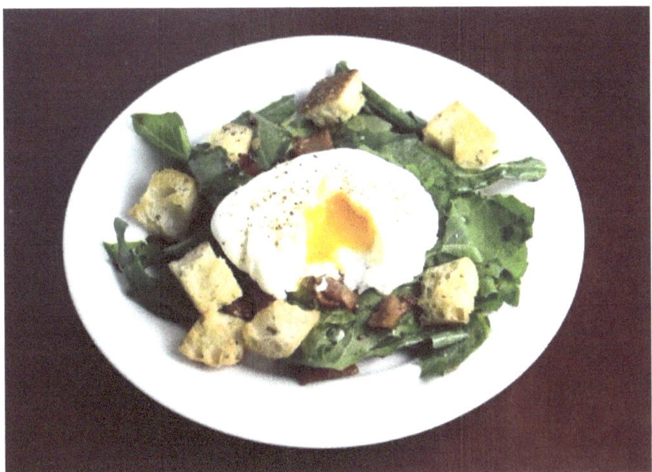

Serves: 2

Preparation Time: 10 minutes

Ingredients

- 2 eggs
- 2 cups Lettuce
- 1 cucumber
- 1 cup micro cress
- 1 cup Greek yogurt
- 2 tbsp. curry powder
- 2 tbsp. oil
- 2 tbsp. cayenne pepper
- 1 tsp. nigella seeds

Directions

1. Add eggs into the bowl.
2. Mix lettuce, cucumber, micro cress, cayenne pepper and nigella seeds.
3. Add oil and yogurt.
4. Mix well.
5. Chill in fridge for 10 minutes.
6. When ready, serve!

Wholegrain Salad with Shallot Yoghurt Dressing

This sophisticated salad is packed with wholegrain goodness.

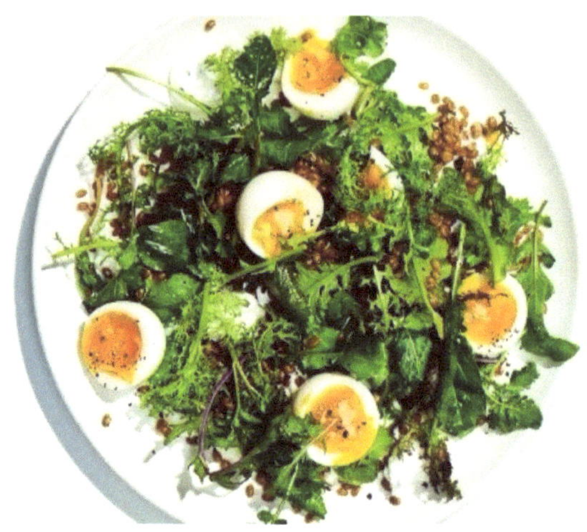

Serves: 4

Preparation Time: 1 hour 15 mins

Ingredients

- ½ cup rye berries
- 1 shallot (chopped)
- ¾ cup full-fat Greek yogurt
- 2 tbsp. fresh mint (chopped)
- 1 tbsp. freshly squeezed lemon juice
- Sea salt and black pepper (to taste)
- 6 cups salad greens
- 4 eggs soft boiled (halved)

Directions

1. Bring a large pot of salted water to a boil. Toss in the rye berries and cook for just over an hour, or until tender.
2. Drain away the water and allow to cool.
3. In a small bowl, combine the shallots, Greek yogurt, chopped mint and half of the lemon juice.
4. Stir well and season with sea salt and black pepper.
5. Add the salad greens and cooled rye berries to a large serving bowl. Pour over the remaining lemon juice and toss well.
6. Arrange the halved soft-boiled eggs on top and drizzle over the yogurt dressing.
7. Serve, enjoy!

Egg, Potato, and Tuna Salad

This is a recipe to get creative with; steamed broccoli and asparagus are good add-ins.

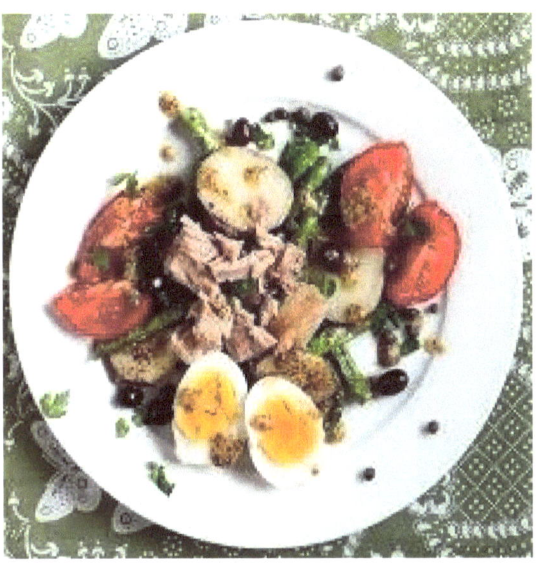

Serves: 4

Preparation Time: 20 minutes

Ingredients

- 8 ounces small new potatoes (red or white)
- 4 large eggs, hard-cooked, peeled, and quartered
- one 6-ounce can tuna, drained
- 1 rib celery, chopped
- ¼ cup chopped red onion or scallion
- 1 tbsp. chopped fresh parsley
- 1 tablespoon minced fresh dill
- 1 teaspoon grated lemon zest
- ½ teaspoon kosher salt
- ¼ teaspoon freshly ground black pepper

For the dressing

- 1 tbsp. mayonnaise
- 1 tbsp. lemon juice
- 1 tbsp. extra-virgin olive oil
- 1 tbsp. coarse mustard
- 1 teaspoon granulated sugar

Directions

1. Bring a medium pot of water to a boil and boil the potatoes until just tender.
2. Let cool, and then cut into quarters.

3. Put the potatoes and eggs in a bowl.
4. Flake the tuna and add to the bowl. Gently mix these ingredients. Add the celery, onion, parsley, dill, and lemon zest and toss gently.
5. Add the salt and pepper, and stir once more.
6. Whisk the dressing ingredients together until well blended.
7. Pour over the salad and toss to coat.

Chapter 4. Egg Soup

Lemon Soup

An extremely flavorsome Greek soup. Serve with warm crusty bread with eggs for a delicious lunch.

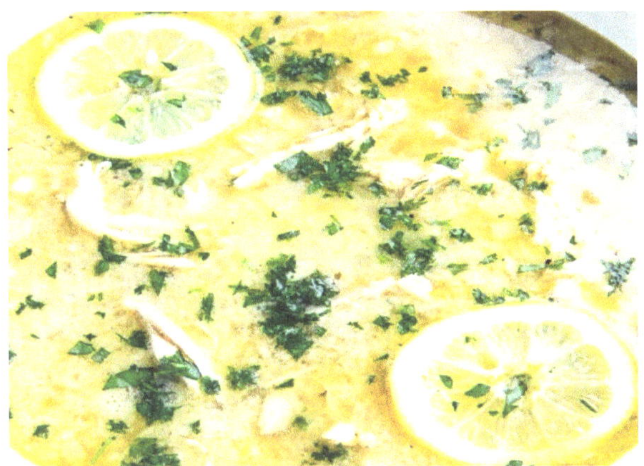

Serves: 6-8

Preparation Time: 1 hour 20 minutes

Ingredients

- 1 (35-40 ounce) fresh chicken
- 1 red onion (peeled)
- 5 cups cold water
- Salt and black pepper (for seasoning)
- 6-7 ounces plain rice
- 2 large eggs (at room temperature)
- Juice of 1 lemon

Directions

1. Place the chicken in a large deep saucepan. Add the red onion, peeled but still whole. Add enough cold water to completely cover the bird. Season well with salt and pepper.
2. Place the saucepan over a high heat and bring to a boil. Reduce heat to medium and cover with a tightly fitting lid. Gently boil the chicken for approx. 60-70 minutes. (The chicken is cooked when the meat falls away from the carcass and juices run clear). Using a slatted spoon, skim off any surface foam from the water.
3. Remove the chicken from the pan and set aside.
4. Drain the broth and pour into a medium saucepan. Add the rice and season with salt and pepper. Bring to boil.
5. In the meantime, pull the chicken meat away from the bones and discard any skin. Cut the meat into bite size cubes.

6. Crack the 2 eggs into a clean large bowl. Whisk until foamy. Add the lemon juice and continue to whisk. Next, add a ladleful of the hot soup to the egg-juice mixture and whisk. Repeat this process until all the soup has been transferred to the bowl. The eggs should now be warm. Pour the mixture into the saucepan. Stir the soup, cover with a lid, and leave for 4-5 minutes.
7. Serve warm, sprinkled with the chicken cubes and seasoned with pepper.

Curry Egg Drop Soup

Egg drop soup, packed with vitamins and minerals, is a great cure-all for colds and sniffles.

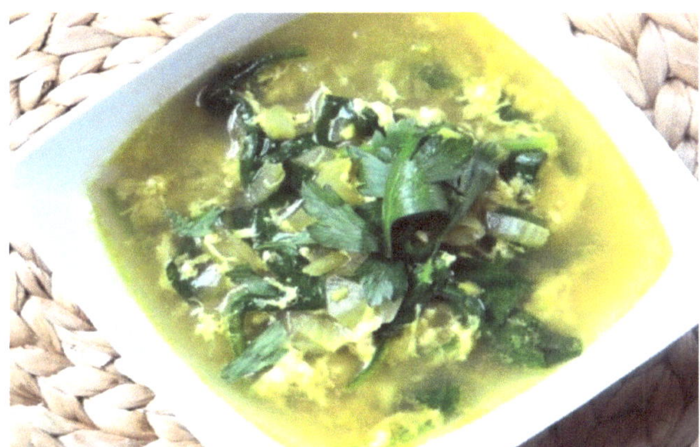

Serves: 2

Preparation Time: 15 minutes

Ingredients

- 1 tbsp. olive oil
- 1 yellow onion (finely chopped)
- 3 garlic cloves
- 1 small piece ginger (peeled, chopped)
- 1 tsp curry powder
- 4 cups vegetable stock
- salt and black pepper (to taste)
- 3 cups fresh spinach
- 2 medium eggs (beaten)
- fresh chopped parsley (to garnish)

Directions

1. Heat the oil in a pot. When hot, add in the onions and sauté for 5 minutes, until softened.
2. Add in the garlic and ginger, sauté for another couple of minutes.
3. Sprinkle in the curry powder.
4. Pour in the vegetable stock, stir well and then season with salt and pepper. Turn the heat to a gentle simmer.
5. Toss in the spinach. After 30 seconds, take a wooden spoon and start to stir the soup, using large circular motions.
6. Continue to stir while you pour the beaten egg into the pot in a steady stream.
7. Ladle immediately into warm bowl and top with fresh parsley.

Italian Egg Soup

Although reminiscent of the classic Italian soup stracciatella, you won't find my recipe in an Italian cookbook. It's something I came up with that uses Italian ingredients in a way that satisfies me. This soup is thick, deeply flavorful, and easy to prepare, and it uses ingredients that I always have on hand.

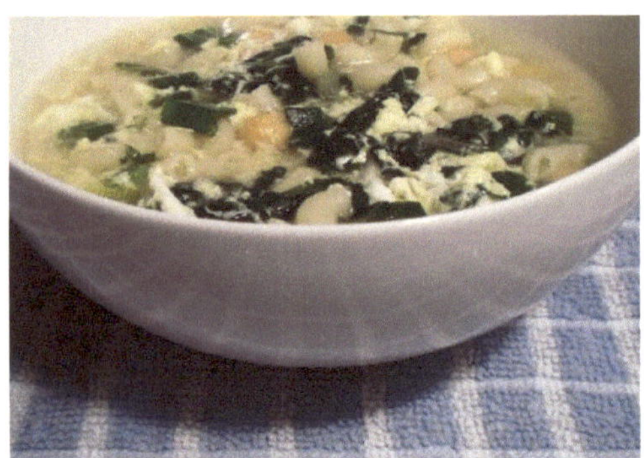

Serves: 6
Preparation Time: 30 minutes

Ingredients

- 6 ounces baby spinach
- 3 tablespoons extra-virgin olive oil
- ½ cup cubed pancetta
- 1 cup chopped onion
- 2 cloves garlic, minced
- ⅓ cup arborio rice
- 6 cups chicken broth
- ¼ cup grated Romano cheese
- 4 large eggs
- kosher salt
- freshly ground black pepper
- crushed hot red pepper flakes

Directions

1. Wash the spinach (even if the bag says "washed"). Discard any mushy leaves. Heat the olive oil in a large pot. Toss in the pancetta and onion, and cook until the pancetta begins to brown and crisp and the onion softens and turns golden. Add the garlic and cook for a few minutes more.
2. Add the spinach to the pot and cook for about 2 minutes, until wilted. Stir in the rice.
3. Pour in the broth and bring to a simmer. Cover and cook at a low simmer for 20 minutes.

4. Using a fork, stir the cheese and eggs together in a bowl until well combined. Take the pot off the heat and, if desired, pour the soup into a serving tureen. Immediately stir in the egg-cheese mixture. It will cook when it hits the hot soup.
5. Taste and season with salt and pepper if necessary (this will depend on the saltiness of the broth).
6. Sprinkle with hot red pepper flakes.

Spanish Garlic Soup

This soup has the big flavors and full body that are perfect for a winter dinner. It is finished in the oven like French onion soup, but in this case, instead of melted cheese, there is an egg poached on the surface.

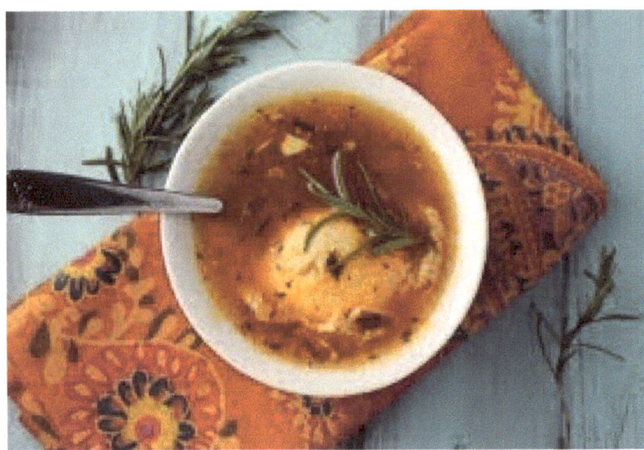

Serves: 4

Preparation Time: 25 minutes

Ingredients

- 3 tablespoons olive oil
- 6 cloves garlic, sliced
- 1 teaspoon sweet paprika
- ½ teaspoon cumin
- ⅛ teaspoon saffron
- 4 crusty bread slices
- chicken broth
- salt
- black pepper
- 4 eggs
- parsley

Directions

1. Heat the olive oil in a large pot. Add the garlic and cook over low heat for about 10 minutes.
2. Add the ingredients.
3. Put the bread in the seasoned oil and toast on both sides.
4. Mix the broth in carefully over the bread.
5. Season with the salt and pepper. Bring the broth to a boil and then immediately lower the heat to a low simmer. If the soup boils too rapidly, the bread will break apart.
6. Preheat the oven to 400 F. Put 4 ovenproof soup bowls on a baking sheet. Ladle the soup and a slice of bread into each bowl.

7. Crack an egg into each soup bowl. Slide the baking sheet into the oven (it's much easier than handling each bowl) and bake until the yolks are set, 8 to 10 minutes.
8. Sprinkle each serving with the cilantro.

Egg Drop Soup

This is a lighter, home-style recipe. It is very easy to prepare and makes a wonderful late-night supper when you come home tired and think there is nothing in the house.

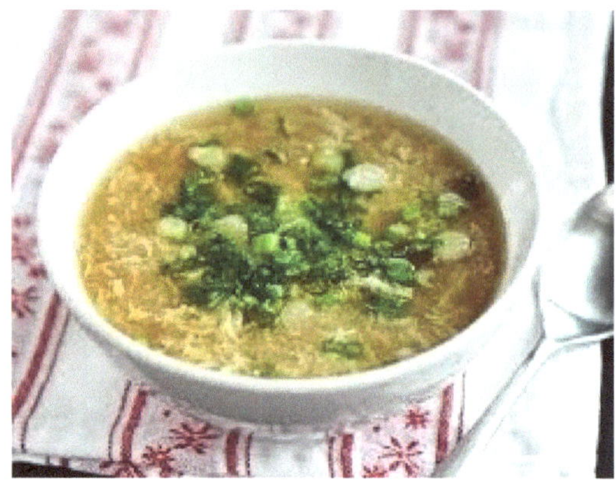

Serves: 4

Preparation Time: 20 minutes

Ingredients

- 4 cups chicken broth
- 2 slices peeled fresh ginger (about 1 by ⅛ inch)
- 2 cloves garlic, smashed and peeled
- 1 teaspoon kosher salt
- 2 large eggs
- 1 teaspoon dry sherry
- 2 scallions, sliced, using all the white and most of the green
- 2 tablespoons chopped fresh cilantro

Directions

1. Bring the broth, ginger, and garlic to a boil in a large pot. Lower the heat and simmer gently for 5 minutes.
2. Discard the ginger and garlic. Stir in the salt. Lower the heat to a very low simmer.
3. In a small bowl, mix the eggs and sherry with a fork.
4. Pour the eggs into the soup in a slow, steady stream, swirling them into the soup. The eggs will set in strands.
5. Remove from the heat and stir in the scallions and cilantro.
6. Serve immediately. Enjoy!

Chapter 5. Sauce (Mayonnaise, Egg Butter, Hollandaise Sauce)

The only mayonnaise recipe you'll ever need. Now you'll never have to buy preservative packed mayo from the store again.

Ultimate Mayo

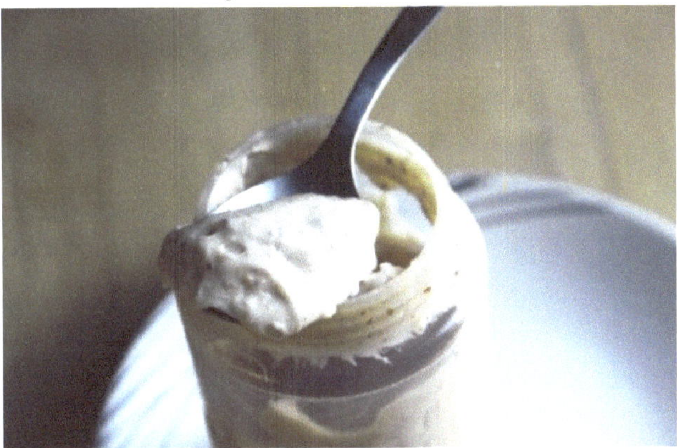

Serves: 12 - 14

Preparation Time: 15 minutes

Ingredients

- 2 egg yolks
- ¾ cup vegetable oil
- 1½ tbsp. white wine vinegar
- ½ tsp Kosher salt
- ½ tsp black pepper

Directions

1. Add the egg yolks to a bowl. Use an electric whisk to beat the yolks until frothy.
2. Drizzle 2 ½ tsp of the canola in slowly, whilst continuously whisking for another 40 seconds.
3. Add the remaining oil, vinegar salt and black pepper.
4. Whisk until all ingredients are well combined.
5. Store, covered, in the refrigerator for 2-3 days.

Eggs Florentine

A variation of Eggs Benedicts but this dish substitutes bacon with spinach. The secret to the success of this recipe lies in the sauce. It needs to cook slowly and gently.

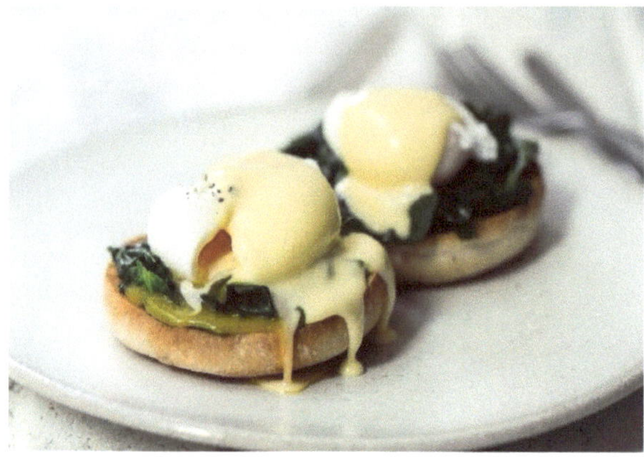

Serves: 4

Preparation Time: 55 minutes

Ingredients

- Hollandaise sauce
- 4 egg yolks
- 2 tbsp. fresh lime and lemon juice
- 1 tbsp. cold water
- 1/8 tsp salt
- 2 pinches white pepper (freshly ground)
- Pinch cayenne pepper
- Eggs Florentine
- 2 sticks unsalted butter (melted)
- 4 white English muffins (split, toasted)
- 3 tsp unsalted butter (softened)
- 4 cups loosely packed baby spinach leaves
- 8 medium eggs

Directions

1. To make the sauce: Set a large heatproof bowl over a saucepan of water, barely simmering. Make sure that the base of the bowl is larger than the saucepan and therefore does not touch the water in the pan.
2. In the heatproof bowl combine the egg yolks, lime and lemon juice, and cold water. Whisk continually until the mixture thickens. Continue to whisk for a further minute, making sure to remove the bowl from the pan immediately when you see it thickening. Season with salt, pepper and cayenne.
3. Use an aerator attached to a hand blender and blend the mixture, while at the same time gently pouring the sticks of melted butter in a fine stream. It should take about 2-3 minutes for the mixtures to be incorporated. Taste and season as

needed. Cover and keep the sauce warm on a very low heat until you are ready to serve.

4. Spread a thin layer of butter (2 teaspoons in total) on both sides of each muffin.
5. In a frying pan on a medium heat, melt 1 teaspoon of butter. Add the spinach to the pan and fry until it wilts slightly, about 2-3 minutes. Keep the spinach warm.
6. Add ½" cold water to an egg poaching pan, and on a medium heat bring to a slow simmer. Spray the cups with cooking spray and carefully break an egg into each greased cup. Cover the pan and poach until the whites are formed and yolks glazed but still runny, this should take around 3-4 minutes depending on your preference.
7. Transfer the cooked eggs to a warm dinner plate and repeat until all the eggs have been used.
8. Lay 2 buttered muffin halves on 4 dinner plates. Top the base of each muffin with spinach, a poached egg and hollandaise sauce.
9. Serve immediately!

Egg Mayo Fill

Easy and simple recipe of egg to get yourself some protein daily!

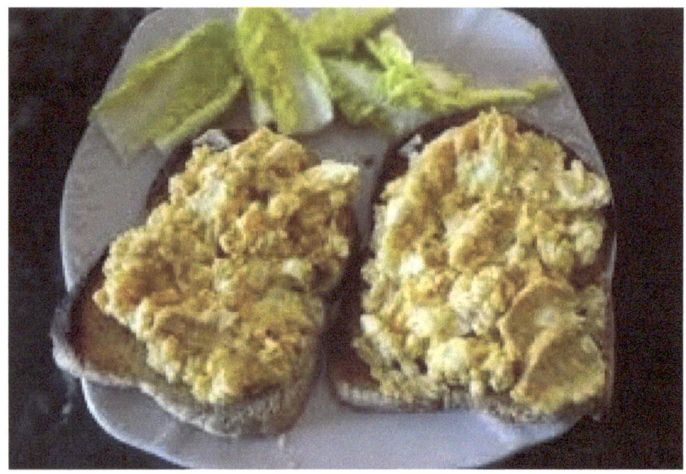

Serves: 2

Preparation Time: 15 minutes

Ingredients

- Boiled eggs–3
- Egg mayonnaise–2 tbsp.
- Fresh chives–2 tbsp.
- Dijon mustard–2 tbsp.

Directions

1. Add the boil yolk into the bowl and keep the white part of egg separate.
2. Mash the yolk into the bowl.
3. Add mayonnaise, chives and mustard.
4. When ready, fill the empty part of white egg and enjoy!

Mayonnaise

If you've never had homemade mayonnaise, how good it is will surprise you. The color will, too: It's yellow, not white like the jarred version. There are few lunches better than a homegrown-tomato and bacon sandwich made with fresh mayonnaise.

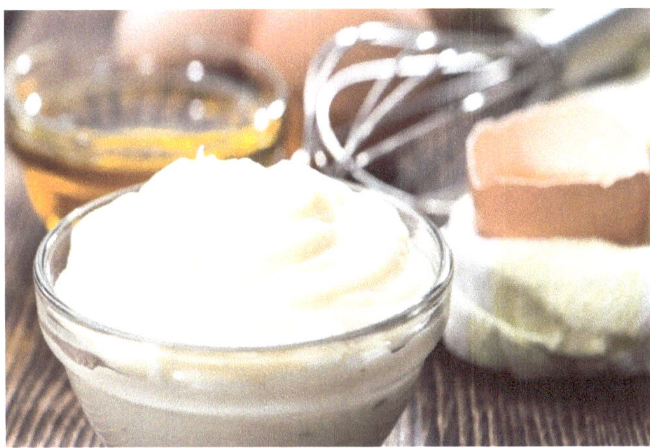

Makes 1 cup

Ingredients

- 1 large egg
- 2 egg yolks
- 1 teaspoon Dijon mustard
- 1 tablespoon lemon juice
- ½ teaspoon kosher salt
- ⅛ teaspoon freshly ground black pepper
- ¾ cup vegetable oil

Directions

1. Put the egg, egg yolks, mustard, lemon juice, salt, and pepper in a medium bowl and whisk until thick.
2. While whisking constantly, add the oil in a slow, steady stream and continue to whisk until thick.
3. The mayonnaise will begin to separate after about a day.
4. A brisk whisking will thicken it up again.
5. Use within 3 days.

Aioli

Aioli is garlicky, lemony homemade mayonnaise. It is rich, smooth, and pungent. It is great as a dip for crudités, a sauce for steamed vegetables, a spread for sandwiches or a dipping.

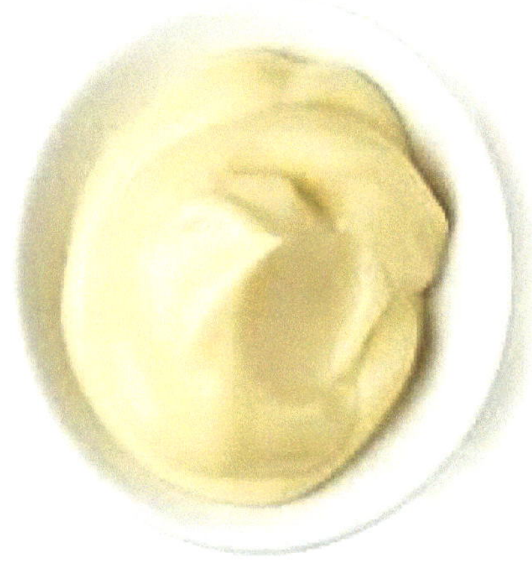

Makes 1 cup

Ingredients

- 4 cloves garlic, peeled
- ½ teaspoon kosher salt
- 2 egg yolks
- 1 teaspoon Dijon mustard
- ¼ teaspoon freshly ground white or black pepper
- 3 teaspoons lemon juice
- 1 cup extra-virgin olive oil

Directions

1. Using a chef's knife, mash and mince the garlic with the salt until you get a smooth paste.
2. In a small bowl, whisk the garlic paste and egg yolks.
3. Add the mustard and pepper, and whisk until smooth. Whisk in 1 teaspoon of the lemon juice.
4. Add half of the oil in a slow, steady stream, whisking vigorously until thick.
5. Stir in the remaining 2 teaspoons lemon juice, and then finish whisking in the oil.
6. Enjoy!

Chapter 6. Pasta Doughs (Basic Egg Pasta, Chinese Egg Noodles)

Classic Creamy Carbonara

The eggs make for a thick, creamy sauce. Combined with bacon and plenty of parmesan, this is a truly indulgent pasta.

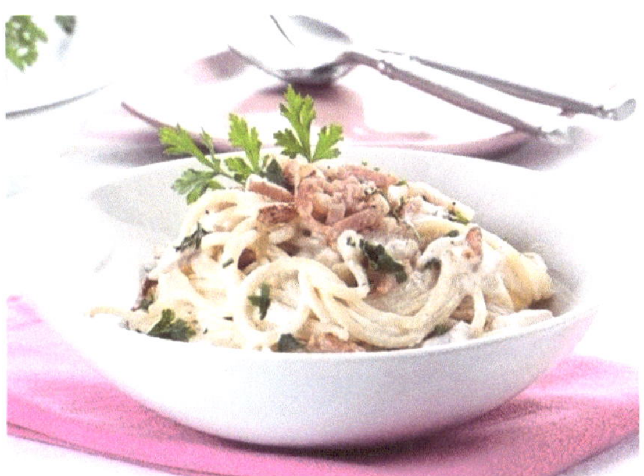

Serves: 3-4

Preparation Time: 30 minutes

Ingredients

- 2 tbsp. sea salt
- 1 pound spaghetti
- 1 tbsp. olive oil
- ½ pound bacon (chopped)
- ½ white onion (chopped)
- 5 medium eggs
- ¼ cup whole milk
- ¼ cup shredded Parmesan
- 1 tsp black pepper
- Fresh chopped parsley (for garnish)

Directions

1. Take a large pot, fill with water and sprinkle with salt. Bring to a roaring boil. When boiling, add in the spaghetti and cook until al dente.
2. In the meantime, take a clean skillet and heat the olive oil. When 'popping' toss in the bacon pieces and sauté for a few minutes before draining any excess fat and adding in the onion. Sauté until the onions have softened and bacon is crispy.
3. In a clean bowl, beat the eggs and whisk in the milk, shredded Parmesan and pepper. Set to one side.

4. Drain the water from the pot of pasta and return the pot with the spaghetti to the heat. While continuously stirring, pour in the milk/egg mixture.
5. Toss in the bacon and onions. Continue to stir for 3-4 minutes until heated through.
6. Use a spaghetti fork to divide the pasta equally into warmed bowls.
7. Sprinkle with fresh chopped parsley and serve immediately.

Egg Spaghetti

If you feel like you are lacking in vitamins then this is full meal for you to have during the day.

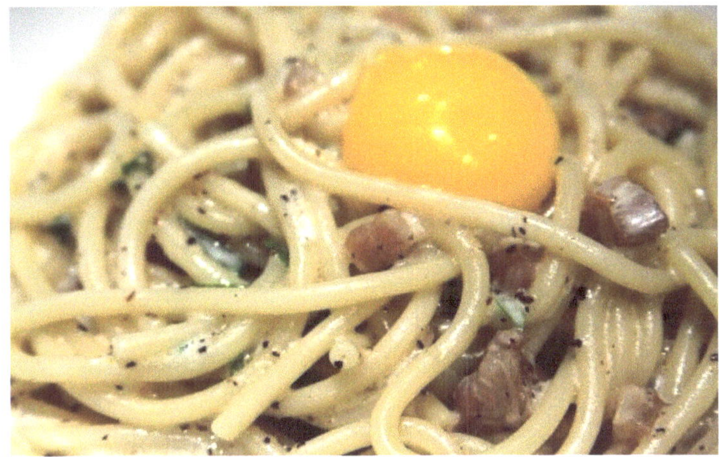

Serves: 2

Preparation Time: 15 minutes

Ingredients

- Asparagus – 2
- Onion(chopped) – 1
- Garlic cloves(chopped) – 2
- Fresh herbs – 2 tbsp.
- Lemon juice – 2 tbsp.
- Butter – 2 tbsp.
- Breadcrumbs – 2 cups
- Spaghetti – 1 pack
- Eggs – 4

Directions

1. Boil the spaghetti and keep aside when done.
2. Add butter into the pot and cook on low heat.
3. Add asparagus, onion, garlic, herbs, lemon juice, breadcrumbs and eggs.
4. Cook for 10 minutes.
5. When ready, mix both spaghetti and mixture to enjoy.

Lemon Chile Rigatoni with Grated Egg Yolk

Yes, you really can grate egg yolks! And what's more, they're the perfect garnish for buttery lemon chile rigatoni.

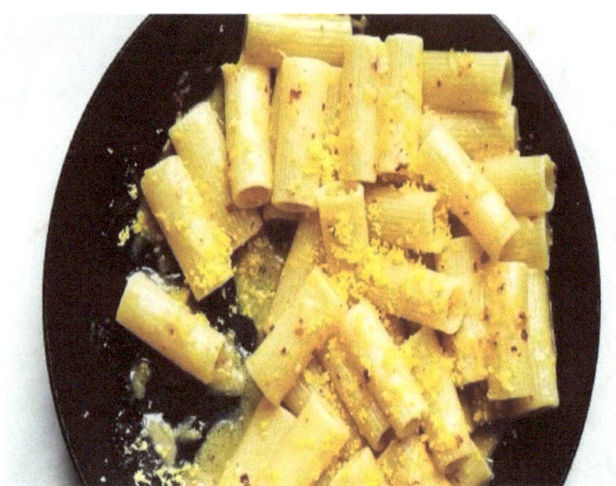

Serves: 4

Preparation Time: 25 minutes

Ingredients

- Sea salt
- 12 ounces dried rigatoni
- 4 large hardboiled eggs
- 8 tbsp. butter
- 2 tsp lemon zest (grated)
- 4 tbsp. freshly squeezed lemon juice
- ½ tsp red Chile pepper flakes (crushed)
- Black pepper (to taste)
- ½ cup Pecorino cheese (grated)

Directions

1. Salt a large pot of water and bring to a boil. Toss in the rigatoni and cook until very al dente.
2. In the meantime, separate the yolks from the hard boiled eggs and discard the whites.
3. Gently grate the yolks into a small bowl and set aside.
4. Drain the pasta into a bowl, setting aside 1½ cups of the cooking water.
5. In a skillet over med-high heat, melt ¾ of the butter and sauté the lemon zest, juice and crushed red pepper flakes.
6. Add the pasta to the skillet along with the reserved cooking water. Cook for 4-5 minutes until the sauce thickens.
7. Season with black pepper and extra salt if necessary.
8. Sprinkle the cheese over the pasta and add in the remaining butter.
9. Toss until the cheese and butter melt and coat the pasta.

10. Spoon the pasta evenly into warmed bowls and finish with a sprinkle of grated egg yolk.
11. Enjoy!

Local Egg Noodle Casserole

At less than 500 calories per serving, this casserole is a great way to enjoy a nutritious and healthy meal.

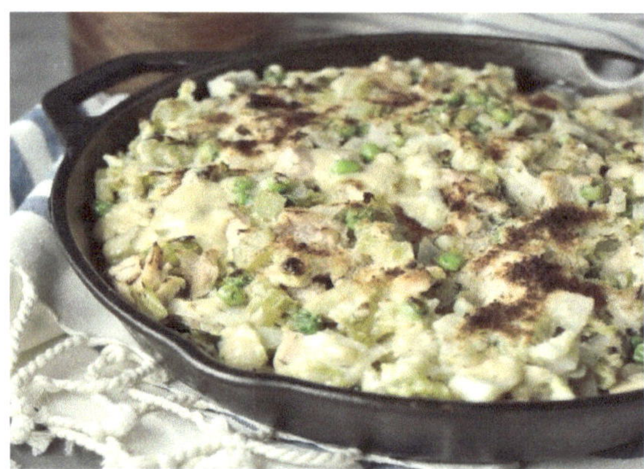

Serves: 4

Preparation Time: 40 minutes

Ingredients

- 3 cups dry broad egg noodles (cooked)
- 2 cups pasta sauce
- 1 cup low fat cottage cheese
- 8 eggs (hardboiled, peeled, sliced)
- 1 cup low-fat mozzarella cheese (grated)
- 2 tbsp. fresh Parmesan cheese (grated)

Directions

1. Preheat the main oven to 350 F.
2. Lightly coat a 2 quart casserole dish with cooking spray.
3. Add 1½ cups of cooked noodles, 1 cup of pasta sauce, ½ cup of cottage cheese, ½ of the sliced egg and ½ cup of grated mozzarella to the dish.
4. Repeat the layer. Scatter Parmesan cheese over the top of the casserole and completely cover with foil.
5. Transfer to the preheated oven and bake for 15 minutes. Remove the foil and cook for a further 10-12 minutes, until the cheese is bubbling.

Delicious Pasta

This pasta meal is really healthy with vegetable and chicken. Addition of egg on the top of pasta will increase their taste and flavor.

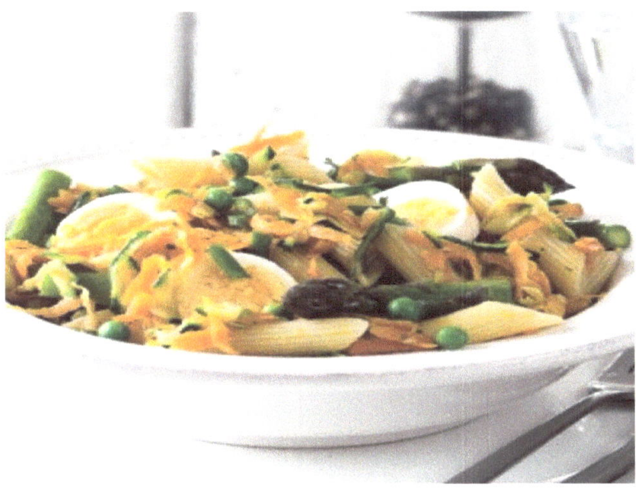

Serves: 4

Preparation Time: 35 minutes

Ingredients

- 500 ml chicken stock
- 250 g rice (long grain)
- 300 g turkey (cooked and diced)
- 250 g baby spinach
- 2 shredded carrot
- 1 teaspoon sesame oil (toasted)
- 1 teaspoon sesame seed (toasted)
- 2 tablespoons vegetable oil
- 4 eggs
- 2 tablespoons chili sauce

Directions

1. Take a large pan and pour chicken stock in it. Let this stock boil and add the chicken and pasta into it. Let it boil again and cook for almost 12 to 15 minutes.
2. Put rice and turkey in a bowl and keep it aside.
3. In the meantime, place spinach in one colander and pour hot water on spinach to make it lightly wilt. Keep carrots and spinach in separate bowls, but sprinkle sesame seeds and oil on both bowls.
4. Cover your cooked rice and keep them aside. Take a cooking pan and heat some vegetable oil on high heat.
5. Fry eggs to make them crispy and roughly round.
6. Take serving bowls and spoon rice into bowls. Arrange carrots and spinach on the top.

7. Top each bowl with chilli sauce and fried eggs.
8. Serve hot!

And one more important recipe … The recipe for a joyful life!

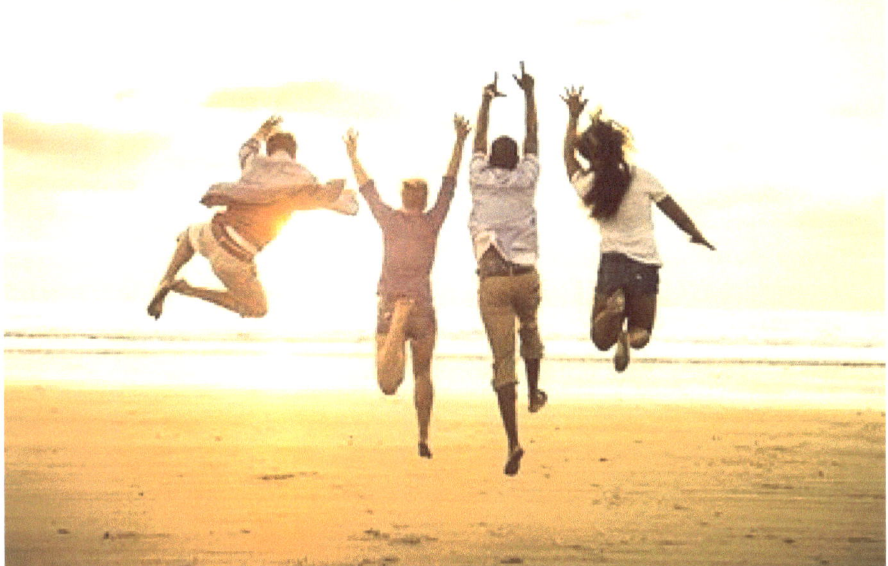

Serves: *all your family*

Cooking Time: *a few minutes every day*

Ingredients

- good mood
- positive thinking

Directions

- *Make small surprises for your loved ones*
- *Do charity work*
- *More often do your favorite thing*
- *Spend more time with children and the elderly*
- *Go in for sports*
- *Read books*
- *Learn the languages*
- *More walking*
- *Do exercises*
- *Throw away unnecessary things from home*
- *Plan an interesting weekend*
- *Take photos*
- *Smile more often*
- *Hug your loved ones*
- *Meditate*

There have been a lot of concerns that people think eggs increase cholesterol but they do not if you eat them within limits. The cholesterol levels get high when you have salt intake or when you are having too many oily foods. There is no saturated fat associated with the eggs so you can have them without any worry.
It gives you a healthy heart in future run. You can promote various healthy activities associated with eggs such as if you come back from a workout and after half an hour you consume egg, you will see how much energy you will gain in just a few minutes. It helps you in brain development as well with the baby during pregnancy; you will be able to have an increase in blood along with energy levels. There won't be any digestive problems and your diet will be balanced as well.

Eggs are necessity for the body because of the level of protein it contains cannot be found anywhere else. There is no food item which can be a substitute for one another so if you think you can avoid eggs and gain the similar nutrients from somewhere else, that won't be happening.
We need nutrients to survive healthy on daily basis which is why there are numerous recipes available for you in this book so you can try them at home at your convenience. If you think you have been feeling weak then it is the time you go and purchase eggs and cook anything out of it. The best part about eggs is that it never loses its nutrients no matter how you cook it so do not worry about that but only regarding your health.

Thank you for purchasing this book!

I hope you will apply the acquired knowledge productively!